I0427186

# CKD Stage 4

## Cookbook for Seniors

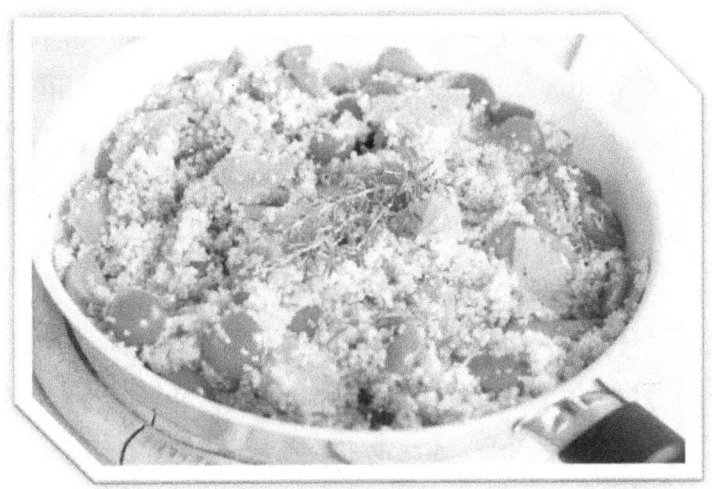

50 Nutritious Low Sodium and Low Potassium
Recipes to manage Chronic Kidney Disease

**Alvin Lewis**

# Copyright © 2024 by Alvin Lewis.

**All rights reserved.**

No part of this publication may be reproduced, distributed, or transmitted in any form or by any means, including photocopying, recording, or other electronic or mechanical methods, without the prior written permission of the publisher, except in the case of brief quotations embodied in critical reviews and certain other noncommercial uses permitted by copyright law.

## Disclaimer

The information and recipes provided in this cookbook are intended for general informational purposes only. The author and publisher are not responsible for any adverse effects or consequences resulting from the use or misuse of the content contained herein. Readers are advised to consult with a qualified healthcare professional or nutritionist before making significant dietary changes, especially if they have existing health conditions or concerns.

# Table of Contents

# More Books from the Author

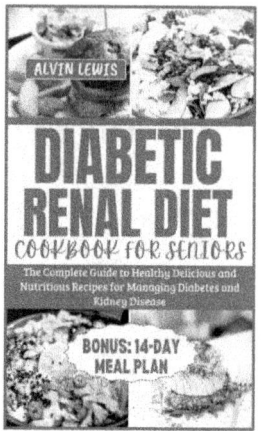

**Diabetic Renal Diet Cookbook for Senior**

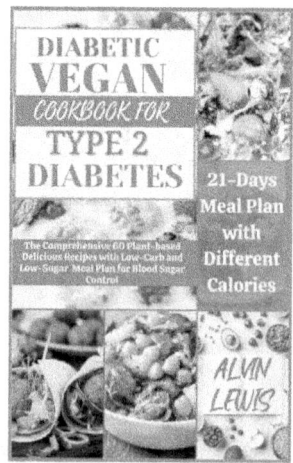

**Diabetic Vegan Cookbook for Type 2 Diabetes**

# Introduction

Margaret, an old woman used to reside in a peaceful town surrounded by meandering streams and rolling hills. At the age of 65, Margaret received the difficult diagnosis of Stage 4 Chronic Kidney Disease (CKD). But instead of giving up, she embarked on a journey to reclaim her health through the transformative power of the right diet.

Margaret, a retired school teacher, who is renowned for her tenacity and resolve, accepted the diagnosis with optimism. Equipped with knowledge from her physician and motivated by the notion that diet could serve as her ally, she embarked on a quest to comprehend the nuances of a diet that is suitable for her kidneys.

Margaret turned her tiny kitchen into a haven of hope, experimenting with different products and cooking methods. She replaced processed foods with fresh fruits and vegetables, carefully monitored her protein intake, and became adept at creating flavorful meals without relying on excessive salt.

Margaret embraced the challenge of adapting traditional recipes to align with her newfound dietary principles.

Margaret's kitchen developed into a colorful, soothing oasis with every day that went by. She enjoyed cooking meals that satisfied her palate as well as nourishing her body. Her dedication to her well-being went beyond what she ate; she participated in moderate workouts, cultivated awareness, and surrounded herself with uplifting people.

Months later, Margaret's dedication bore fruit. Her regular check-ups revealed improvements in her kidney function that astounded her healthcare team. As the once-daunting CKD Stage 4 started to recede, Margaret's vitality increased. She turned into a ray of hope for many in her community dealing with related medical issues.

Margaret's tale resonated with people of all ages throughout the area. Her experience demonstrated the capacity for transformation offered by a kidney-friendly, well-balanced diet as well as the resiliency of the human spirit. Margaret's CKD Stage 4 was reversed during this treatment, and she also developed a renewed enthusiasm for life that was evident in everything she did.

Margaret became a living example of the significant positive effects that mindful eating and lifestyle modifications may have on health as she told others about her experience. Her kitchen, once a haven for culinary experimenting, now served as a reminder that it's never too late to take control of one's health and appreciate life's bounty and a symbol of triumph over hardship.

Welcome to the CKD Stage 4 Cookbook for Seniors, a gastronomic adventure designed to empower and transform lives. We urge you to explore a path to wellness on the pages that follow, where a healthy diet can be a ray of hope for people facing the challenges of Stage 4 Chronic Kidney Disease (CKD).

This cookbook is not just a collection of recipes; it's a comprehensive guide that addresses the complexities of chronic kidney disease (CKD), from comprehending its complexities to creating delectable meals that nourish the body and the spirit. Come discover how to transform every meal into a celebration of resilience and overall well-being as we explore the art of cooking for kidney health.

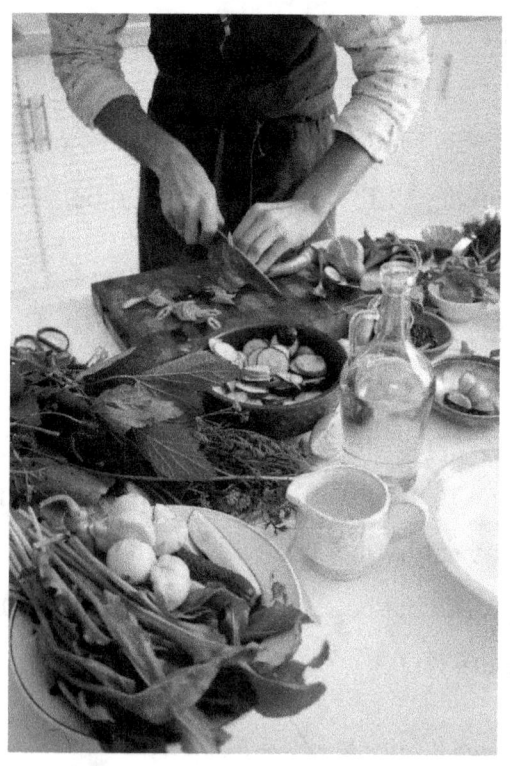

# Chapter 1: Understanding CKD Stage 4

## Overview of Chronic Kidney Disease (CKD) Stage 4

Chronic Kidney Disease (CKD) Stage 4 is a critical stage that requires care and proactive management. With the kidneys functioning at a filtration rate of 15 to 29 milliliters per minute, this stage denotes a substantial deterioration in kidney function. Investigating CKD Stage 4's main features, including its causes, symptoms, and effects on general health, is essential to understanding the condition.

### Causes and Risk Factors

Stage 4 CKD frequently results from the advancement of prior stages or underlying illnesses. The leading culprits that progressively impair renal function are diabetes and hypertension. Genetic predispositions, autoimmune diseases, and recurring kidney infections are other factors.

Identifying and addressing these root causes are fundamental steps in managing CKD Stage 4.

## Symptoms and Warning Signs

Symptoms appear when kidney function deteriorates, emphasizing the urgency of prompt treatment. Common indications include fatigue, fluid retention, and changes in urine frequency and color. Anemia and other problems, such as worsening hypertension, could occur. It is imperative to consistently observe these indicators in order to assess the advancement of Stage 4 CKD.

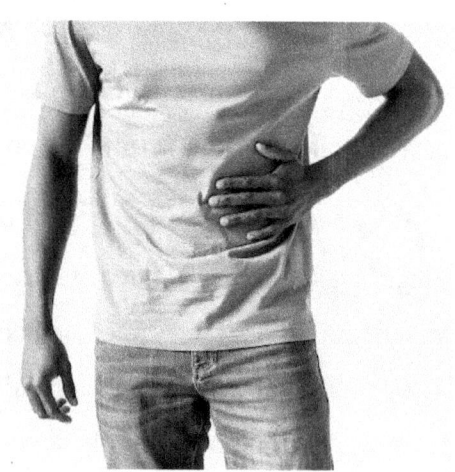

# Importance of Early Detection and Treatment

Effective care of Stage 4 CKD depends on early identification. Routine screenings, including blood tests measuring creatinine and glomerular filtration rate (GFR), enable healthcare professionals to diagnose and intervene promptly. In order to create a thorough treatment plan, patient, caregiver, and healthcare provider collaboration is essential.

Realizing that you have Stage 4 CKD encourages a comprehensive approach to lifestyle changes. Dietary modifications, such as restricted sodium intake, regulated protein intake, and attentive hydration, are helpful. Medication management becomes tailored to address complications such as hypertension and anemia. Reducing stress, giving up smoking, and engaging in regular exercise all improve general wellbeing.

Being aware of Stage 4 CKD is the first step toward enabling people to take control of their health. Through adopting a holistic viewpoint that encompasses mental, physical, and lifestyle elements, individuals can move through this stage with fortitude and make decisions that improve their quality of life.

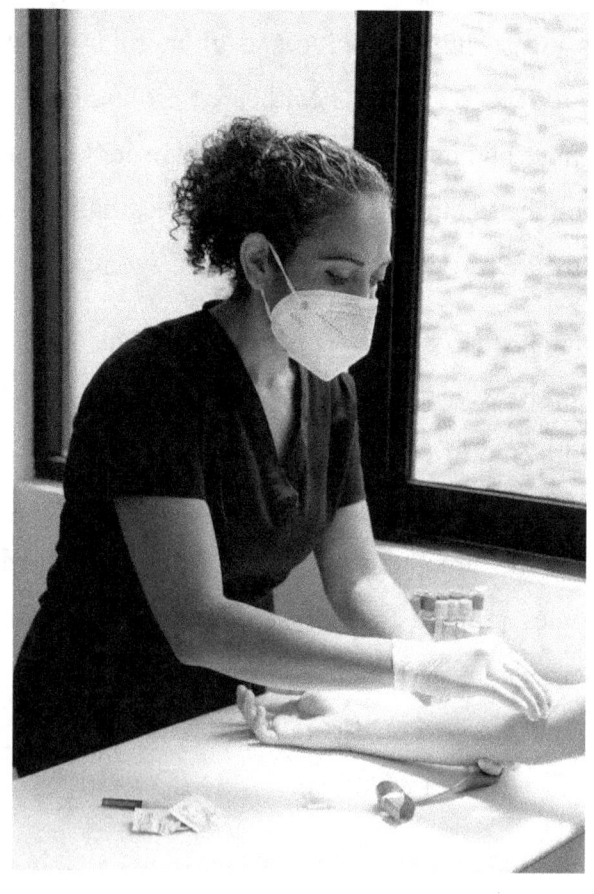

# Chapter 2: The CKD Stage 4 Friendly Diet

## Overview of the CKD Stage 4 Diet

A careful nutritional strategy is required for managing symptoms, promoting general health, and potentially slowing the progression of the condition in Chronic Kidney Disease (CKD) Stage 4. Crafting a CKD Stage 4 diet involves balancing nutritional needs while addressing the challenges posed by compromised kidney function.

Proper nutrition is crucial in CKD Stage 4. In order to limit the burden on compromised kidneys and maintain the provision of vital amino acids, it becomes imperative to regulate protein consumption. It's critical to keep an eye on potassium and phosphorus levels since imbalances might lead to difficulties. To address bone health and anemia frequently linked to chronic kidney disease (CKD), an adequate diet of calcium, vitamin D, and iron is essential.

## Portion Control and Meal Frequency

Portion management is crucial in Stage 4 CKD to control waste product accumulation. Regularly eating smaller meals helps to keep the metabolic state steady, which lessens the strain on the kidneys. Tailoring portion amounts to suit individual requirements, physical activity levels, and medical background is essential for making the CKD Stage 4 diet uniquely tailored.

## Foods to Eat for CKD Stage 4

Choosing foods that promote renal function and provide essential nutrients is part of creating a CKD Stage 4 diet. The following is a list of foods that can be a part of this particular diet:

### 1. Superior Sources of Protein

*Lean Meats:* Skinless poultry and lean beef.

*Fish:* Fatty fish rich in omega-3 fatty acid such as salmon, trout, and others

*Eggs:* A flexible and high-protein food choice.

*Plant-Based Proteins:* Tofu, legumes, and beans provide alternative protein sources.

## 2. Nutritious Carbohydrates

*Whole Grains*: Oats, brown rice, quinoa, and whole wheat pasta provide long-lasting energy.

*Fruits:* Berries, apples, and grapes in moderation to reduce potassium content.

*Vegetables:* Low-potassium options include cabbage, cauliflower, and green beans.

## 3. Essential Fats

*Olive oil:* A good source of monounsaturated fats for the heart.

*Avocados*: Low in phosphorus and Rich in good fats.

*Nuts and Seeds:* For extra nutrition, try almonds, flaxseeds, and chia seeds.

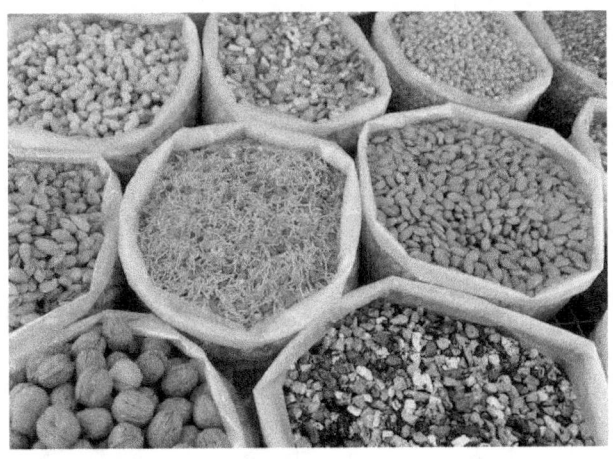

### 4. Dairy Alternatives:

**Low-Phosphorus Dairy:** If dairy is included, choose modest servings of low-phosphorus dairy products like milk and yogurt.

*Non-Dairy Substitutes:* Rice, coconut, or fortified almond milk can serve as an appropriate substitute.

### 5. Using Herbs and Spices in Cooking

*Fresh Herbs:* Parsley, cilantro, basil, and other herbs to add taste without added sodium.

*Spices:* Ginger, turmeric, and cumin can improve flavor without adding sodium intake.

### 6. Vegetables and Fruits

*Berries:* For antioxidants, try blueberries, strawberries, and raspberries.

*Apples:* A low-potassium fruit that can be enjoyed in numerous ways.

*Bell Peppers:* A colorful, low-potassium vegetable rich in vitamins.

*Cabbage:* A cruciferous vegetable with health advantages and low potassium.

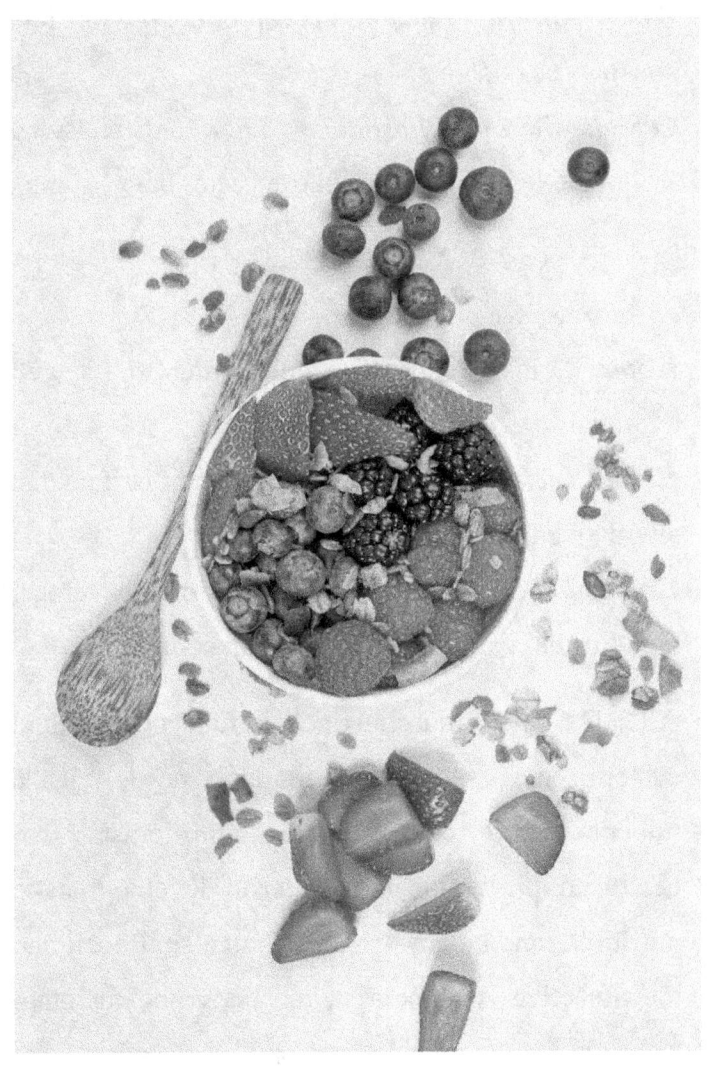

### 7. Bread and Cereal

*Whole Grain Bread:* Select products with less phosphorus contents.

*Cereals with Low Phosphorus:* Look for cereals that are made especially for those who have kidney problems.

### 8. Beverages

*Water:* Drink plenty of simple water to be well hydrated.

*Herbal Teas:* For variation, try these non-caffeinated alternatives.

*Homemade Smoothies:* For a nutrient-rich beverage, blend fruits, vegetables, and protein sources.

A CKD Stage 4 diet must be carefully planned and customized based on individual needs. It is imperative to consult with nutritionists and healthcare professionals in order to develop a tasty, nutritious, and kidney-friendly food plan. Recall that the objective is to nourish the body and maintain kidney function, and moderation is essential.

# Foods to Avoid for Stage 4 CKD

Making thoughtful dietary decisions is essential for managing Stage 4 Chronic Kidney Disease (CKD) in order to reduce the burden on the kidneys. Here is a thorough list of items to stay away from when following the CKD Stage 4 diet:

## 1. High Sodium Foods

*Processed Meats:* Sausage, deli meats, and bacon frequently have high sodium content.

*Canned Soups:* Prepackaged soups may contain a lot of sodium.

*Packaged Snacks:* Foods like crackers, chips, and pretzels may contribute to excessive sodium intake.

## 2. Foods High in Potassium

*Bananas:* A potassium-rich fruit that needs to be consumed in moderation.

*Oranges and Orange juice:* Rich in phosphate and potassium.

*Tomatoes and Tomato Products:* Potassium-rich sauces and ketchup included.

### 3. Foods High in Phosphorus

*Dairy Products:* Yogurt, cheese, and milk all contain a lot of phosphorus.

*Nuts and Seeds:* Nuts like sunflower, peanut, and almond seeds can be rich sources of phosphorus.

*Chocolate:* Phosphorus and potassium are both present.

### 4. Foods High in Oxalate

*Swiss chard and spinach:* Rich in oxalates, which may aggravate kidney stones.

*Beets:* Contain both oxalates and potassium.

*Chocolate and Tea:* Should be consumed in moderation due to oxalate content.

### 5. Processed Convenience Foods

*Frozen Meals:* Frequently rich in phosphorus and sodium.

*Fast food:* Typically high in sodium, it can lead to an unhealthy diet.

# Chapter 3: Breakfast Ideas

## 1. Quinoa Breakfast Bowl

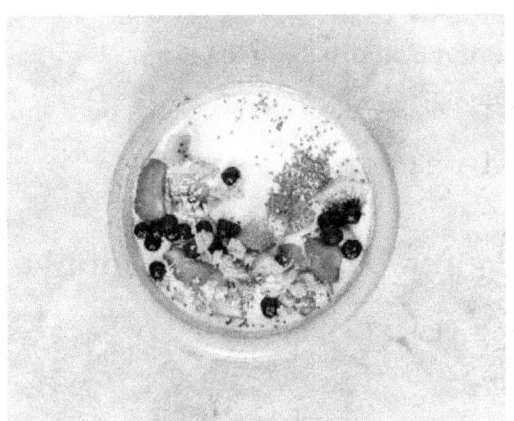

**Cooking Time: 20 minutes**

*Ingredients:*

- 1/4 cup sliced strawberries
- 1/2 cup rinsed quinoa
- 1 cup water
- 1 teaspoon honey
- 1 tablespoon chopped almonds

*Guidelines:*

1. In a saucepan, combine quinoa and water. Bring to a boil, then reduce heat and simmer for 15 minutes.

2. After the quinoa is cooked, transfer it to a bowl and fluff it with a fork.

3. Top with almonds, strawberries, and drizzle of honey.

**Nutritional Benefits:** Quinoa is a protein-rich grain, and strawberries offer antioxidants and vitamin C. Almonds contribute healthy fats.

## 2. Egg and Vegetable Scramble

**Cooking Time: 10 minutes**

*Ingredients:*

- 2 eggs
- 1 tablespoon olive oil
- 1/4 cup chopped zucchini
- 1/4 cup diced bell peppers
- To taste, add salt and pepper.

*Guidelines:*

1. In a pan over medium heat, warm up the olive oil.

2. Sauté zucchini and bell peppers until tender.

3. Whisk the eggs and transfer them to the pan. Scramble until cooked.

4. Add pepper and salt for seasoning.

**Nutritional Benefits:** Bell peppers and zucchini contribute vitamins and minerals, while eggs give high-quality protein.

# 3. Oatmeal with Berries and Almond Milk

**Cooking Time: 5 minutes**

*Ingredients:*

- 1/4 cup mixed berries
- 1/2 cup rolled oats
- 1 cup unsweetened almond milk
- 1 tablespoon chia seeds

*Guidelines:*

1. Cook the rolled oats in almond milk as directed on the packet.

2. Top with mixed berries and chia seeds.

**Nutritional Benefits:** Berries provide antioxidants, and oats provide fiber. Chia seeds supplement with omega-3 fats.

## 4. Greek Yogurt Parfait

**Cooking Time: 5 minutes**

*Ingredients:*

- 1/2 cup plain Greek yogurt
- 1/4 cup (low-phosphorus) granola
- 1/4 cup peach slices
- 1 tablespoon honey

*Guidelines:*

1. Arrange sliced peaches, Greek yogurt, and granola in a glass.

2. Drizzle with honey.

**Nutritional Benefits:** Greek yogurt provides protein, while peaches offer vitamins and fiber. Granola adds crunch.

## 5. Sweet Potato Hash

**Cooking Time: 15 minutes**

*Ingredients:*

- 1 tablespoon olive oil
- 1/2 teaspoon dried thyme
- 1/2 cup diced sweet potatoes

- 1/4 cup chopped onions
- 1/4 cup diced bell peppers.

**Guidelines:**

1. In a pan over medium heat, warm up the olive oil.

2. Add bell peppers, onions, and sweet potatoes. Cook until golden and softened.

3. Sprinkle dried thyme on top.

**Nutritional Benefits:** Sweet potatoes are rich in vitamins, and bell peppers provide additional vitamins and antioxidants.

# 6. Cottage Cheese and Pineapple Bowl

**Cooking Time: 5 minutes**

**Ingredients:**

- 1 tablespoon shredded coconut
- 1/2 cup of low-fat cottage cheese
- 1/2 cup of diced pineapple

*Guidelines:*

1. In a bowl, mix together cottage cheese and diced pineapple.

2. Add shredded coconut to top.

**Nutritional Benefits:** Pineapple offers sweetness and vitamin C, while cottage cheese is a healthy source of protein.

## 7. Whole Wheat Toast with Avocado and Poached Egg

**Cooking Time: 10 minutes**

*Ingredients:*

- 1/4 mashed avocado
- 1 slice whole wheat bread
- 1 poached egg
- To taste, add salt and pepper.

*Guidelines:*

1. Toast the whole wheat bread.

2. Top the toast with mashed avocado.

3. Add a poached egg on top and season with pepper and salt.

**Nutritional Benefits:** Whole wheat provides fiber, and avocado offers healthy fats. The poached egg adds protein.

# 8. Blueberry Smoothie Bowl

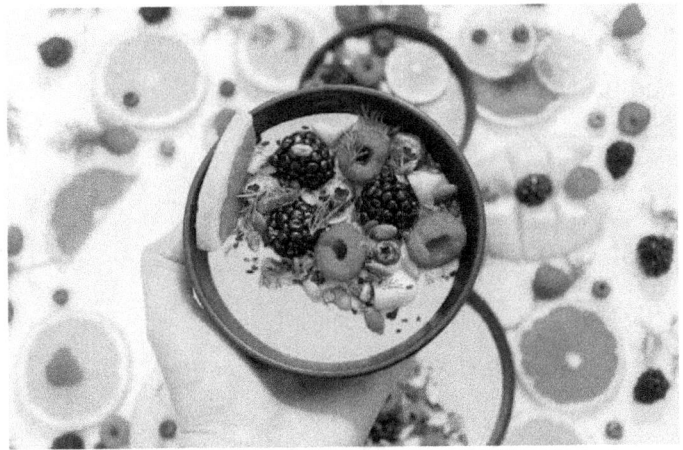

**Cooking Time: 5 minutes**

*Ingredients:*

- 1/2 banana
- 1 cup frozen blueberries
- 1 tablespoon chia seeds
- 1 tablespoon almond butter

- 1/2 cup unsweetened almond milk

*Guidelines:*

1. Blend banana, almond milk, and frozen blueberries in a blender until smooth.

2. Transfer to a bowl and garnish with almond butter and chia seeds.

**Nutritional Benefits:** Blueberries are rich in antioxidants, and almond butter provides healthy fats and protein.

## 9. Ricotta and Berry Stuffed Crepes

**Cooking Time: 15 minutes**

*Ingredients:*

- 1/2 cup ricotta cheese
- 1/4 cup mixed berries
- 1 teaspoon honey
- 2 whole grain crepes

*Guidelines:*

1. Spread ricotta cheese on crepes.

2. Add mixed berries and drizzle with honey.

3. Fold the crepes and serve.

**Nutritional Benefits:** Ricotta contributes protein, and berries offer vitamins and antioxidants.

# 10. Spinach and Feta Omelette

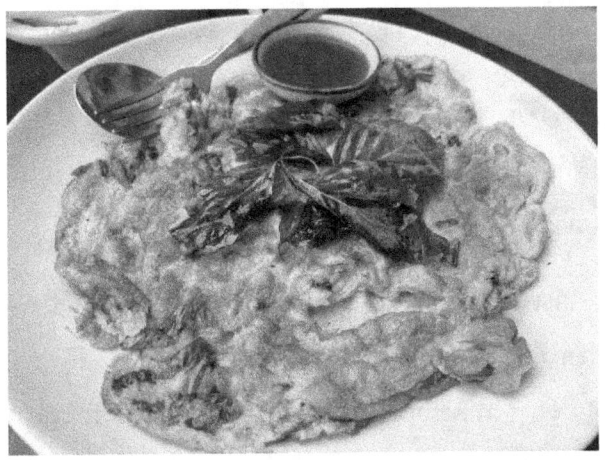

**Cooking Time: 8 minutes**

*Ingredients:*

- Two eggs
- 1 tablespoon crumbled feta cheese
- 1/4 tablespoon chopped spinach
- 1 teaspoon olive oil

## Guidelines:

1. Whisk eggs in a bowl.

2. In a pan over medium heat, warm the olive oil.

3. Pour eggs into the pan, add chopped spinach and feta cheese.

4. Fold the omelette after cooking until the eggs are set.

**Nutritional Benefits:** Feta adds flavor and calcium, and spinach is high in vitamins and iron.

These tasty and kidney-friendly CKD Stage 4 breakfast alternatives are made to meet the dietary requirements of seniors. Adapt serving sizes to meet specific nutritional needs, and seek the advice of medical professionals for individualized recommendations at all times.

# Chapter 4: Sumptuous Lunches

## 1. Salmon and Quinoa Salad

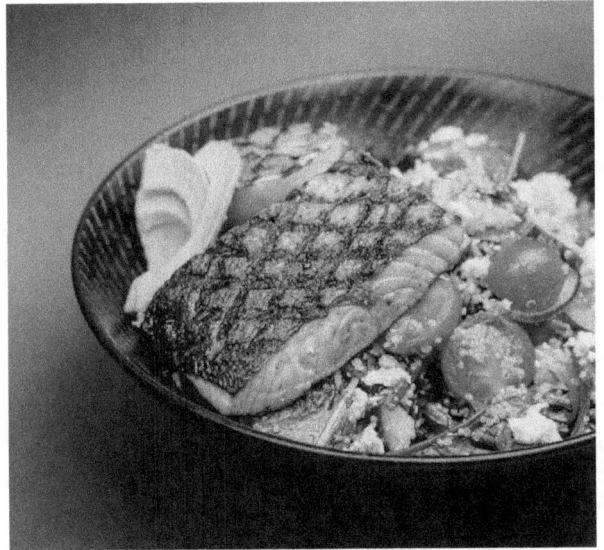

**Cooking Time: 15 minutes**

*Ingredients:*

- 4 ounces of grilled salmon
- 1 cup mixed greens
- 1/2 cup cooked quinoa
- 1/4 cup chopped cherry tomatoes

- 1 tablespoon lemon dressing and olive oil

*Guidelines:*

1. Grill salmon until cooked.

2. Combine cherry tomatoes, mixed greens, and cooked quinoa.

3. Top with grilled salmon and drizzle with olive oil and lemon dressing.

**Nutritional Benefits:** Quinoa gives fiber and protein, and salmon offers omega-3 fatty acids. Tomatoes and greens provide vitamins.

# 2. Turkey and Avocado Wrap

**Cooking Time: 5 minutes**

*Ingredients:*

- 1 whole wheat tortilla
- 3 ounces sliced turkey breast
- 1/4 sliced avocado
- 1/2 cup shredded lettuce
- 1 tablespoon low-fat mayo

*Guidelines:*

1. Spread out the whole wheat tortilla.

2. Spread mayo, then top with lettuce, avocado, and turkey slices.

3. Roll the tortilla into a wrap.

**Nutritional Benefits:** Turkey is a lean protein source, and avocado provides healthy fats and fiber.

# 3. Vegetable Stir-Fry with Tofu

**Cooking Time: 15 minutes**

*Ingredients:*

- 1 cup mixed stir-fry vegetables (broccoli, snap peas, bell peppers)
- 1/2 cup cubed tofu
- 1 tablespoon (low-sodium) soy sauce
- 1 tsp. sesame oil
- 1/2 cup brown rice, cooked

*Guidelines:*

1. Heat sesame oil in a skillet over medium heat, stir-fry tofu until golden.

2. Add mixed vegetables and cook until softened.

3. Stir in soy sauce and serve over cooked brown rice.

**Nutritional Benefits:** Mixed vegetables include vitamins and minerals, and tofu provides plant-based protein.

## 4. Mediterranean Chickpea Salad

**Cooking Time: 10 minutes**

*Ingredients:*

- 1/4 cup sliced cucumbers
- 1/2 cup canned, drained chickpeas
- 1/4 cup halved cherry tomatoes
- 2 tablespoons crumbled feta cheese
- 1 tablespoon balsamic vinegar dressing
- 1 tablespoon olive oil

*Guidelines:*

1. In a bowl, mix together chickpeas, cucumbers, cherry tomatoes, and feta.

2. Drizzle with balsamic vinegar dressing and olive oil.

**Nutritional Benefits:** Vegetables and feta offer taste and vitamins, while chickpeas are high in protein and fiber.

## 5. Chicken and Vegetable Kebabs

### Cooking Time: 20 minutes

*Ingredients:*

- 4 ounces cubed grilled chicken
- 1/2 cup onions and bell peppers,
- 1/2 cup cherry tomatoes
- 1 tablespoon lemon marinade
- 1 tablespoon olive oil
- 1/2 cup quinoa, cooked

*Guidelines:*

1. Marinate chicken in olive oil and lemon marinade.

2. Put vegetables and chicken onto skewers.

3. Grill chicken until cooked. Serve on top of cooked quinoa.

**Nutritional Benefits:** Chicken offers protein, and vegetables provide vitamins. Quinoa adds protein and fiber.

## 6. Egg Salad Lettuce Wraps

**Cooking Time: 15 minutes (including boiling eggs)**

*Ingredients:*

- 2 hard-boiled eggs, diced
- 2 tablespoons low-fat mayo
- 1 tablespoon Dijon mustard
- 1/4 cup chopped celery
- Lettuce leaves to wrap

*Guidelines*:

1. In a bowl, combine chopped eggs, mustard, mayo, and celery.

2. Transfer the egg salad onto the lettuce leaves and wrap.

**Nutritional Benefits:** Celery adds crunch and vitamins, and eggs provide protein.

## 7. Shrimp and Asparagus Stir-Fry

**Cooking Time: 15 minutes**

*Ingredients:*

- 4 ounces peeled and deveined shrimp

- 1/2 cup asparagus, cut into pieces
- 1 tablespoon soy sauce (low-sodium)
- 1 tablespoon of olive oil
- 1/2 cup quinoa, cooked

*Guidelines:*

1. Heat olive oil in a pan, then stir-fry shrimp until pink.

2. Add asparagus then cook until softened.

3. Stir in soy sauce and serve over cooked quinoa.

**Nutritional Benefits:** Asparagus offers vitamins and fiber, and shrimp is a low-fat source of protein.

# 8. Caprese Salad with Balsamic Glaze

**Cooking Time: 5 minutes**

*Ingredients:*

- 1/2 cup cherry tomatoes, halved
- 1 tablespoon balsamic glaze
- 2 ounces freshly sliced mozzarella
- Fresh basil leaves

*Guidelines:*

1. Layer cherry tomatoes and mozzarella on a plate.

2. Add some fresh basil leaves as a garnish and drizzle with balsamic glaze.

**Nutritional Benefits:** Mozzarella offers calcium and protein, while tomatoes supply vitamins.

## 9. Vegetarian Lentil Soup

**Cooking Time: 30 minutes**

*Ingredients:*

- 1/2 cup dry lentils
- 1/4 cup diced celery and carrots
- 1/4 cup chopped onions
- 1 minced clove garlic
- 1 tablespoon olive oil
- 4 cups vegetable broth (low-sodium)

*Guidelines:*

1. Rinse and set aside lentils.

2. In a pot, sauté onions, carrots, celery, and garlic in olive oil until tender.

3. Add vegetable broth and lentils. Simmer until lentils are softened.

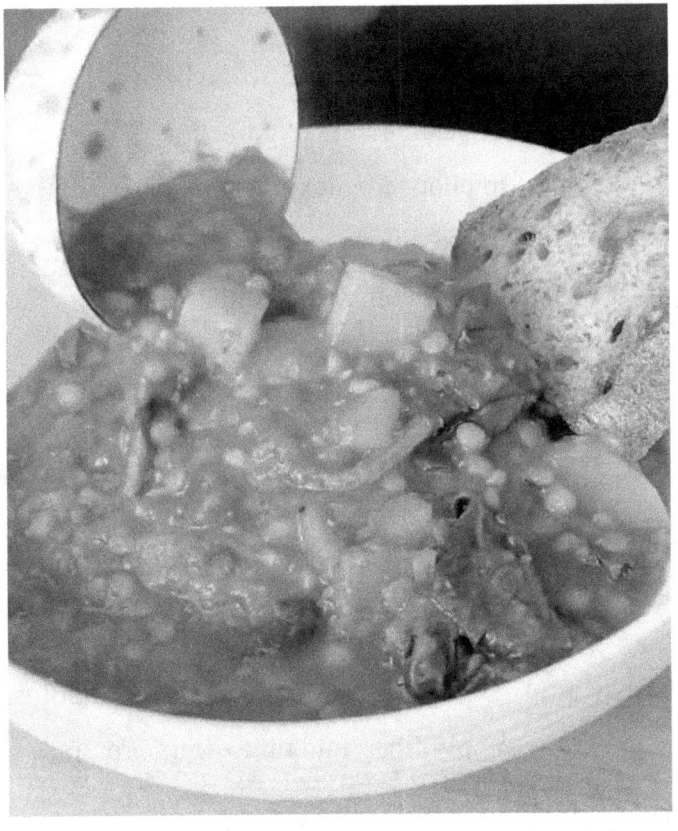

**Nutritional Benefits:** Vegetables contribute vitamins and fiber, while lentils are a good source of plant-based protein.

# 10. Tuna and White Bean Salad

**Cooking Time: 10 minutes**

*Ingredients:*

- 1/2 cup drained canned white beans
- 2 ounces canned tuna, drained
- 1/4 cup chopped cucumbers
- 1/4 cup red onions, diced
- 1 tablespoon lemon dressing
- 1 tablespoon olive oil

*Guidelines:*

1. In a bowl, combine cucumbers, red onions, tuna, and white beans.

2. Drizzle with lemon dressing and olive oil.

**Nutritional Benefits:** Vegetables add vitamins, white beans supply fiber, and tuna offers protein.

These CKD Stage 4 sumptuous lunches are made to be tasty and kidney-friendly, meeting the dietary requirements of seniors. Adjust portion sizes based on individual dietary requirements, and always consult with healthcare professionals for personalized guidance.

# Chapter 5: Dinner Recipes

## 1. Baked Lemon Herb Chicken

**Cooking Time: 30 minutes**

*Ingredients:*

- 1 tablespoon fresh lemon juice
- 1 tablespoon olive oil
- 4 ounces boneless, skinless chicken breast
- 1 teaspoon dried herbs (thyme, rosemary)
- To taste, add salt and pepper.

*Guidelines:*

1. Preheat the oven to 375°F (190°C).

2. Apply salt, pepper, lemon juice, herbs, and olive oil to the chicken.

3. Bake for 25 to 30 minutes, or until chicken is thoroughly cooked.

**Nutritional Benefits:** Chicken is a lean protein source, and herbs add flavor without excess sodium.

## 2. Vegetarian Stir-Fried Tofu and Broccoli

**Cooking Time: 20 minutes**

*Ingredients:*

- 1 cup broccoli florets
- 1/2 cup cubed tofu
- 1 tablespoon (low-sodium) soy sauce
- 1/2 cup cooked brown rice
- 1 tablespoon sesame oil

*Guidelines:*

1. Heat sesame oil in a pan over medium heat and stir-fry the tofu until golden.

2. Add broccoli and cook until softened.

3. Stir in soy sauce and serve over cooked brown rice.

**Nutritional Benefits:** Broccoli contributes vitamins and fiber, while tofu offers plant-based protein.

# 3. Salmon and Vegetable Foil Packets

**Cooking Time: 20 minutes**

*Ingredients:*

- 1/2 cup sliced cherry tomatoes
- 1/2 cup zucchini, sliced
- 1 tablespoon olive oil
- 1 tablespoon lemon juice
- 4 ounces salmon fillet
- Herbs for seasoning (parsley, dill)

*Guidelines:*

1. Preheat the oven to 400°F (200°C).

2. Arrange the salmon onto a foil sheet and surround it with vegetables.

3. Drizzle with olive oil, lemon juice, and herbs.

4. Seal the foil and bake for 20 minutes.

**Nutritional Benefits:** Vegetables provide vitamins and antioxidants, and salmon delivers omega-3 fatty acids.

## 4. Spinach and Feta Stuffed Chicken Breast

**Cooking Time: 30 minutes**

*Ingredients:*

- 4 ounces chicken breast
- 1/4 cup chopped spinach
- 1 tablespoon feta cheese crumbles
- 1 teaspoon olive oil
- Season with salt and pepper

*Guidelines:*

1. Preheat the oven to 375°F (190°C).

2. Create a pocket in the chicken breast and fill it with feta and spinach.

3. Rub with olive oil, season with salt and pepper, and bake for 25-30 minutes.

**Nutritional Benefits:** Chicken is a lean protein source, and spinach adds vitamins. Feta provides flavor.

# 5. Lemon Garlic Shrimp and Asparagus Stir-Fry

**Cooking Time: 15 minutes**

*Ingredients:*

- 4 ounces peeled and deveined shrimp
- 1/2 cup asparagus, chopped
- 1 tablespoon lemon juice
- 1 tablespoon olive oil
- 1 minced garlic clove

*Guidelines:*

1. Heat olive oil in a pan, add shrimp and cook until pink.

2. Add lemon juice, garlic, and asparagus.

3. Stir-fry until the asparagus becomes soft.

**Nutritional Benefits:** Asparagus offers vitamins and fiber, and shrimp is a low-fat source of protein.

## 6. Quinoa and Black Bean Stuffed Bell Peppers

**Cooking Time: 30 minutes**

*Ingredients:*

- 1/2 cup rinsed and drained black beans
- 1/2 cup cooked quinoa
- 1/4 cup diced onions
- 1/4 cup chopped tomatoes
- 1/2 teaspoon cumin
- 1 teaspoon olive oil

*Guidelines:*

1. Preheat the oven to 375°F (190°C).

2. Combine cumin, olive oil, quinoa, black beans, tomatoes, and onions.

3. Stuff mixture with bell peppers and bake for 25 to 30 minutes.

**Nutritional Benefits:** Quinoa offers fiber and protein, while black beans give plant-based protein.

# 7. Lentil and Vegetable Soup

**Cooking Time: 30 minutes**

*Ingredients:*

- 1/2 cup dry lentils
- 1/4 cup diced onions
- 1/4 cup celery, diced
- 1/4 cup carrots, chopped
- 1 minced garlic clove
- 4 cups vegetable broth low-sodium
- 1 tablespoon olive oil

*Guidelines:*

1. Rinse and set aside lentils.

2. Sauté carrots, celery, onions, and garlic in olive oil until tender.

3. Add vegetable broth and lentils. Then simmer until lentils are softened.

**Nutritional Benefits:** Lentils are a good source of plant-based protein, and vegetables provide vitamins and fiber.

## 8. Mushroom and Spinach Omelette

**Cooking Time: 10 minutes**

*Ingredients:*

- 2 eggs
- 1/4 cup of mushroom, sliced
- 1 teaspoon olive oil
- 1/2 cup chopped spinach
- To taste, add salt and pepper.

*Guidelines:s*

1. Whisk eggs in a bowl.

2. Heat olive oil in a pan, sauté mushrooms and spinach until wilted.

3. Pour eggs over the veggies, cook until they are set, and then fold into an omelette.

**Nutritional Benefits:** Protein is provided by eggs, and vitamins are found in spinach. Mushrooms give food a taste.

# 9. Sesame Ginger Chicken Stir-Fry

**Cooking Time: 15 minutes**

*Ingredients:*

- 1/4 cup sliced bell peppers
- 1/2 cup broccoli florets
- 1/4 cup thinly sliced chicken breast
- 1 tablespoon low-sodium soy sauce
- 1 tablespoon sesame oil
- 1 tablespoon grated fresh ginger

*Guidelines:*

1. In a pan heat sesame oil, then stir-fry chicken until done.

2. Add ginger, bell peppers, broccoli, and soy sauce.

3. Sauté until the vegetables are softened.

**Nutritional Benefits:** Vegetables supply vitamins, and chicken is a lean protein source. Ginger enhances taste.

# 10. Caprese Pasta Salad

**Cooking Time: 15 minutes**

*Ingredients:*

- 1/2 cup cooked whole grain pasta
- 1/4 cup halved cherry tomatoes
- 2 oz. diced fresh mozzarella
- Fresh basil leaves
- 1 tsp. balsamic glaze

*Guidelines:*

1. In a bowl, mix cooked pasta, mozzarella, cherry tomatoes, and basil.

2. Drizzle with balsamic glaze.

**Nutritional Benefits:** Whole grain pasta offers fiber, and tomatoes provide vitamins. Mozzarella adds calcium and protein.

These tasty and kidney-friendly CKD Stage 4 Dinners are created to meet the dietary requirements of seniors. Adjust portion sizes based on individual dietary requirements, and always consult with healthcare professionals for personalized guidance.

# Chapter 6: Snacks and Dessert

## 1. Mixed Berry Yogurt Parfait

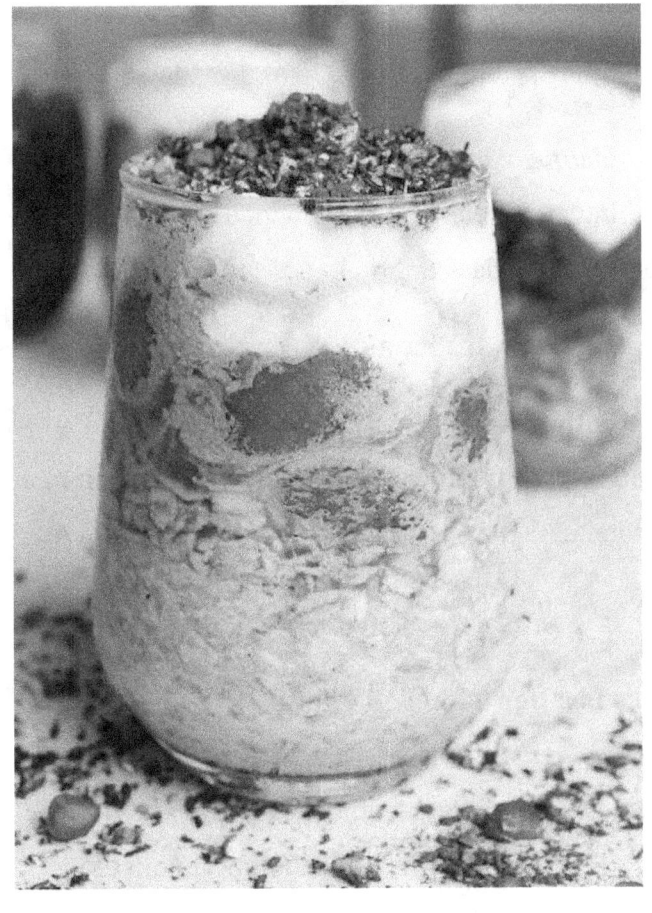

**Prep Time: 5 minutes**

*Ingredients:*

- 1/2 cup low-fat Greek yogurt
- 1/4 cup mixed berries (raspberries, strawberries, and blueberries)
- 1 tablespoon finely chopped nuts (walnuts, almonds)
- 1 tsp. honey

*Guidelines:*

1. Later Greek yogurt, chopped nuts, and mixed berries in a glass or bowl.

2. Drizzle with honey.

**Nutritional Benefits:** Berries supply vitamins and antioxidants, while Greek yogurt offers calcium and protein.

## 2. Cucumber and Hummus Bites

**Preparation Time: 10 minutes**

*Ingredients:*

- 1 medium cucumber, sliced
- 2 tablespoons (low-sodium) hummus

- 1 tablespoon finely chopped fresh dill

*Guidelines:*

1. Arrange cucumber slices on a serving plate.

2. Spoon a small amount of hummus onto each cucumber slice.

3. Add freshly chopped dill as garnish.

**Nutritional Benefits:** Cucumbers are hydrating, and hummus provides protein and healthy fats.

# 3. Baked Apple Slices with Cinnamon

**Preparation Time: 20 minutes**

*Ingredients:*

- 1 medium apple, sliced and cored
- 1/2 teaspoon ground cinnamon
- 1 tsp. honey

*Guidelines:*

1. Preheat the oven to 350°F (175°C).

2. Layer apple slices on a baking sheet.

3. Drizzle with honey and sprinkle with cinnamon.

4. Bake for 15 to 20 minutes, or until the apples are softened.

**Nutritional Benefits:** Cinnamon adds flavor without adding sugar, while apples provide fiber.

## 4. Chia Seed Pudding with Mango

**Preparation Time: 2 hours (plus chilling time)**

*Ingredients:*

- 1/2 cup unsweetened almond milk
- 1 tablespoon shredded coconut
- 2 tablespoons chia seeds
- 1/4 cup diced mango

*Guidelines:*

1. Mix almond milk and chia seeds in a bowl. Then refrigerate for 2 hours or overnight.

2. Stir the chia pudding and sprinkle the shredded coconut and chopped mango over top.

**Nutritional Benefits:** Chia seeds offer omega-3 fatty acids and fiber. Mango adds natural sweetness and vitamins.

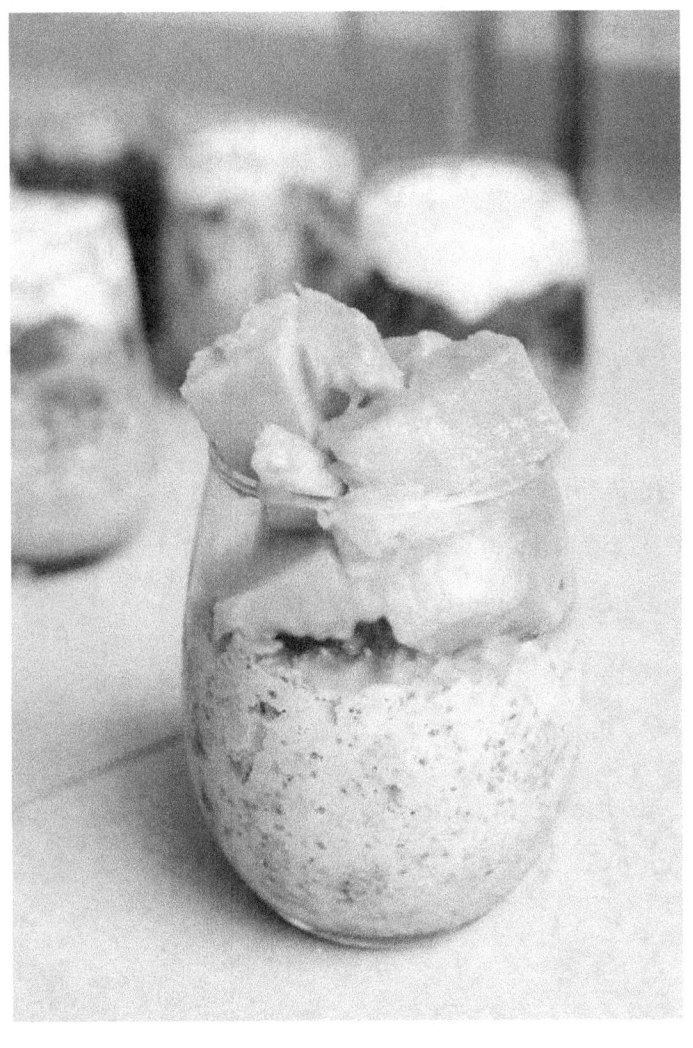

# 5. Avocado and Tomato Salsa

**Preparation Time: 10 minutes**

*Ingredients:*

- 1/2 ripe avocado, diced
- 1/2 cup diced cherry tomatoes
- 1 tablespoon finely chopped red onion
- Fresh cilantro, chopped
- 1 tablespoon lime juice
- To taste, add salt and pepper.

*Guidelines:*

1. Combine diced avocado, cherry tomatoes, red onion, and cilantro in a bowl.

2. Add salt and pepper to taste and drizzle lime juice over the mixture.

**Nutritional Benefits:** Tomatoes supply vitamins and antioxidants, and avocados offer good fats.

# 6. Frozen Banana Bites

**Preparation Time: 1 hour (plus freezing time)**

*Ingredients:*

- 1 banana, sliced into rounds
- 2 teaspoons nut butter (peanut or almond)
- Unsweetened shredded coconut

*Guidelines:*

1. Lightly coat banana slices with nut butter.

2. Sandwich two slices together and roll the edges in shredded coconut.

3. Before serving, place in the freezer for at least 1 hour.

**Nutritional Benefits:** Bananas offer potassium and natural sweetness, while nut butter provides healthy fats.

# 7. Carrot and Hummus Dip

**Preparation Time: 5 minutes**

*Ingredients:*

- 1 cup carrot sticks
- 1 teaspoon sesame seeds

- 2 tablespoons (low-sodium) hummus

*Guidelines:*

1. Arrange carrot sticks on a plate.

2. Garnish with sesame seeds and serve with hummus for dipping.

**Nutritional Benefits:** Hummus supplies protein and good fats. Carrots also include vitamins.

# 8. Cottage Cheese with Pineapple and Mint

**Preparation Time: 5 minutes**

*Ingredients:*

- 1/4 cup diced pineapple
- 1/2 cup low-fat cottage cheese
- Chopped fresh mint leaves

*Guidelines:*

1. Combine diced pineapple and cottage cheese in a bowl.

2. Add some mint leaves as garnish.

**Nutritional Benefits:** Pineapple adds natural sweetness and vitamin C, while cottage cheese offers protein.

# 9. Strawberry Almond Chia Popsicles

**Preparation Time: 4 hours (plus freezing time)**

*Ingredients:*

- 2 tablespoons chia seeds
- 1 cup fresh, hulled strawberries
- 1 cup unsweetened almond milk
- 1 tablespoon honey

*Guidelines:*

1. Blend almond milk, honey, chia seeds, and strawberries in a blender until smooth.

2. Fill the Popsicle molds with the mixture, then freeze for at least 4 hours.

**Nutritional Benefits:** Strawberries offer antioxidants, chia seeds provide omega-3s and fiber, and almond milk is a dairy-free alternative.

# 10. Yogurt and Berries Frozen Bark

**Preparation Time: 3 hours (plus freezing time)**

*Ingredients:*

- 1 cup Greek yogurt (low-fat)
- 1/2 cup mixed berries (raspberries, blueberries)
- 1/4 cup (low-phosphorus) granola
- 1 tbsp. honey

*Guidelines:*

1. In a bowl, mix Greek yogurt and honey.

2. Transfer the mixture onto a parchment-lined tray.

3. Top with granola and mixed berries.

4. Freeze for at least 3 hours, then break into pieces.

**Nutritional Benefits:** Greek yogurt provides protein and calcium, while berries offer antioxidants. Granola adds a crunchy texture.

# Chapter 7: Beverages

## 1. Cucumber Mint Infused Water

**Preparation Time: 2 hours (infusion time)**

*Ingredients:*

- 4 cups water
- 1/2 thinly sliced cucumber
- Fresh mint leaves
- Ice cubes

*Guidelines:*

1. In a pitcher, put cucumber slices and fresh mint leaves.

2. Fill the pitcher with water, refrigerate it for at least 2 two hours.

3. Serve with ice.

**Nutritional Benefits:** Cucumber is hydrating, and mint provides a refreshing flavor without added sugar.

## 2. Berry Citrus Smoothie

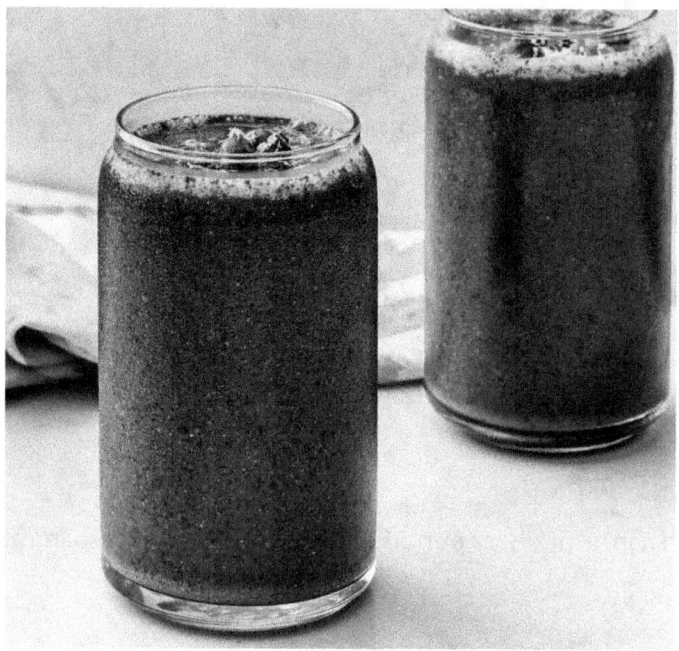

**Preparation Time: 5 minutes**

*Ingredients:*

- 1/2 cup mixed berries (strawberries and blueberries)
- 1/2 banana
- 1/2 cup unsweetened almond
- 1 tablespoon chia seeds
- Ice cubes

## Guidelines:

1. Combine banana, chia seeds, almond milk, and mixed berries in a blender.

2. Blend until smooth.

2. Add ice cubes and blend once more to get the desired consistency.

**Nutritional Benefits:** Almond milk is a dairy-free substitute, berries supply antioxidants, and chia seeds offer fiber and omega-3 fatty acids.

# 3. Turmeric Golden Milk

**Preparation Time: 5 minutes**

## Ingredients:

- 1/2 teaspoon powdered turmeric
- 1 cup unsweetened almond milk
- 1 teaspoon honey
- 1/4 teaspoon cinnamon
- 1/4 teaspoon ginger

## Guidelines:

1. Warm the almond milk, cinnamon, ginger, and turmeric in a saucepan (do not boil).

2. Add honey, stir, and serve.

**Nutritional Benefits:** Almond milk is a low-phosphorus substitute, and turmeric has anti-inflammatory qualities.

## 4. Herbal Tea with Lemon and Fresh Basil

**Preparation Time: 5 minutes**

*Ingredients:*

- 1 cup boiling water
- 1 slice lemon
- 1 herbal tea bag (caffeine-free)
- Fresh basil leaves

*Guidelines:*

1. Steep the herbal tea bag in boiling water for 3-5 minutes.

2. Add some fresh basil leaves and a slice of lemon.

3. Prior to serving, let it cool slightly.

**Nutritional Benefits:** Lemon adds vitamin C, and herbal tea is hydrating. Basil adds a distinct and revitalizing taste.

## 5. Cherry Almond Smoothie

**Preparation Time: 5 minutes**

*Ingredients:*

- 1/2 cup almond milk, unsweetened
- 1/2 cup (fresh or frozen) cherries
- 1/2 tablespoon almond butter
- 1/2 teaspoon vanilla extract
- Ice cubes

*Guidelines:*

1. Blend cherries, vanilla essence, almond butter, and almond milk until smooth.

2. Add ice cubes and blend once more to get the desired consistency.

**Nutritional Benefits:**

Almond butter gives protein and healthy fats, and cherries offer antioxidants.

## 6. Green Tea with Mint and Lemon

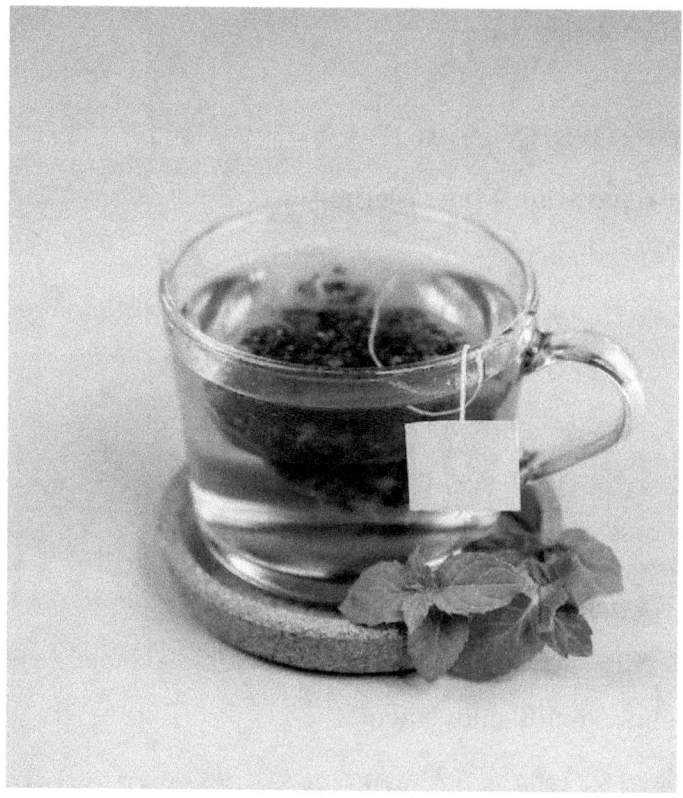

**Preparation Time: 5 minutes**

*Ingredients:*

- 1 green tea bag
- 1 slice lemon
- 1 cup hot water
- Fresh mint leaves

*Guidelines:*

1. Let the green tea bag steep in hot water for 3 to 5 minutes.

2. Add a slice of lemon and some fresh mint leaves.

3. Prior to serving, let it cool slightly.

**Nutritional Benefits:** Green tea is rich in antioxidants, and lemon adds vitamin C. Mint provides a refreshing flavor.

# 7. Pineapple Ginger Sparkler

**Preparation Time: 5 minutes**

*Ingredients:*

- 1/2 cup unsweetened pineapple juice
- 1/2 cup sparkling water
- 1/2 teaspoon grated ginger
- Toppings of fresh pineapple wedges
- Ice cubes

*Guidelines:*

1. Combine grated ginger, sparkling water, and pineapple juice in a glass.

2. Top with fresh pineapple wedges and add ice cubes.

**Nutritional Benefits:** Ginger gives a tangy touch, and pineapple offers natural sweetness and vitamin C.

# 8. Coconut Water with Lime and Basil

**Preparation Time: 5 minutes**

*Ingredients:*

- 1 cup coconut water
- Ice cubes
- Fresh basil leaves
- Juice of 1 lime

*Guidelines:*

1. Combine lime juice and coconut water in a glass.

2. Add the ice cubes and fresh basil leaves.

3. Before serving, give it a gentle stir.

**Nutritional Benefits:** Coconut water is hydrating, lime adds vitamin C, and basil provides a unique herbal flavor.

# 9. Raspberry Basil Iced Tea

**Preparation Time: 10 minutes**

*Ingredients:*

- 1/2 cup fresh raspberries -
- 1 cup boiling water -
- 1 herbal tea bag (free of caffeine).
- Fresh basil leaves -
- Ice cubes

*Guidelines:*

1. Steep the herbal tea bag in boiling water for 3-5 minutes.

2. Add the basil leaves and fresh raspberries.

3. Let it cool, then chill in the refrigerator and serve over ice.

**Nutritional Benefits:** Basil adds a lovely herbal twist, while raspberries contain antioxidants.

# 10. Mango Coconut Smoothie

**Preparation Time: 5 minutes**

*Ingredients:*

- 1/2 cup mango chunks, frozen or fresh
- 1/2 cup coconut water
- 1/4 cup Greek yogurt, plain
- 1 tablespoon shredded coconut
- Ice cubes

*Guidelines:*

1. Combine Mango chunks, Greek yogurt, coconut water, and shredded coconut in a blender.

2. Blend until smooth.

3. Add ice cubes and Blend once more to get the desired consistency

**Nutritional Benefits:** Coconut water is hydrating, and mangos naturally contain vitamins.

# Chapter 8: Meal Planning for Seniors

Seniors with Stage 4 Chronic Kidney Disease must plan their meals carefully in order to effectively manage their illness and preserve their general health. The benefits of meal planning for CKD Stage 4 are explained below:

## CKD Stage 4 Meal Planning Guidelines:

### 1. Limited Sodium Intake:

- Use herbs and spices instead of salt when cooking to increase flavor.

- Opt for fresh, natural foods instead. Because processed and canned meals frequently include significant amounts of sodium,

### 2. Control of Phosphorus:

- Be mindful of foods high in phosphorus, like dairy, nuts, and seeds.

- Reduce your consumption of convenience and processed foods as they may include additives that contain phosphorus.

### 3. Potassium Management:

- Monitor your potassium consumption, emphasizing fruits and vegetables that are low in potassium.

- To lower the potassium level, boil or soak vegetables high in potassium.

### 4. Protein Moderation:

- Modify protein consumption in accordance with personal requirements and medical professionals' advice.

- Choose high-quality sources of protein, such as fish, poultry, eggs, and lean meats.

### 5. Fluid Restriction:

- Adhere to any suggested fluid limitations to prevent the body from being too hydrated.

- Monitor daily fluid intake and include hydrating foods like fruits and vegetables.

### 6. Balanced Nutrient Intake:

- Strive for a diet that is varied in nutrients and well-balanced.

- Focus on whole grains, healthy fats, and a mix of different colored fruits and vegetables.

### 7. Regular Monitoring:

- Use blood tests to regularly check key indicators such as protein, phosphorus, and potassium levels.

- Work closely with healthcare professionals to make adjustments to the meal plan as needed.

# Advantages of Meal Planning in Stage 4 CKD

**1. Disease Management:** Meal planning plays a key role in controlling symptoms like fatigue, edema, and high blood pressure that are linked to Stage 4 CKD.

**2. Nutrient Optimization:** Customized meal plans make sure seniors get the nutrients they need without overdoing them on things their kidneys can't handle.

3. **Preventing Malnutrition:** CKD can lead to malnutrition due to dietary restrictions. Meal planning helps ensure that seniors receive adequate nutrition while adhering to their dietary limitations.

4. **Blood Pressure Control:** Diets low in sodium and potassium can help regulate blood pressure, which is a significant concern for people with chronic kidney disease.

5. **Preventing Further renal Damage:** Controlling phosphorus intake helps preserve overall renal function and avoid further kidney damage.

6. **Improved Quality of Life:** Seniors can have a higher quality of life with more energy and fewer issues by adhering to a specific and well-planned meal plan.

7. **Enhanced Compliance:** Seniors who follow an organized meal plan are more likely to follow dietary recommendations, which improves their general health.

# 14-Days Sample Meal Plan

## Day 1:

*Breakfast:* Scrambled eggs with spinach and feta

- Whole grain toast

*Lunch:* Quinoa and black bean salad with mixed vegetables

- Grilled chicken breast

*Dinner:* Baked salmon with lemon and herbs

*Snack:* Greek yogurt with sliced strawberries

## Day 2:

*Breakfast:* Oatmeal with banana slices and a sprinkle of chia seeds

*Lunch:* Lentil soup with mixed greens salad

*Dinner:* Stir-fried tofu with broccoli and bell peppers

- Mixed berry parfait for dessert

*Snack:* Carrot sticks with hummus

## Day 3:

*Breakfast:* Whole grain waffle with low-potassium fruit compote

*Lunch:* Chicken and vegetable stir-fry with low-sodium soy sauce

*Dinner:* Roasted sweet potatoes

*Snack:* Cottage cheese with pineapple chunks

## Day 4:

*Breakfast:* Smoothie with spinach, berries, almond milk, and a scoop of protein powder

*Lunch:* Grilled chicken Caesar wrap with whole grain tortilla

*Dinner:* Baked lemon herb chicken

*Snack:* Cucumber slices with tzatziki sauce

## Day 5:

*Breakfast:* Whole grain pancakes with sliced peaches and a dollop of low-fat whipped cream
- Orange juice

*Lunch:* Couscous salad with cherry tomatoes and cucumber

*Dinner:* Turkey meatballs with marinara sauce
- Mixed greens salad

*Snack:* Mixed nuts (portion-controlled)

## Day 6:

*Breakfast:* Yogurt parfait with granola and mixed berries

- Green tea

**Lunch:** Quinoa and vegetable stir-fry

**Dinner:** Vegetarian chili with kidney beans and tomatoes

- Baked sweet potato wedges

**Snack:** Rice cake with almond butter

## Day 7:

**Breakfast:** Egg white omelette with mushrooms, tomatoes, and spinach

**Lunch:** Tuna salad with mixed greens

**Dinner:** Grilled vegetable skewers with a balsamic glaze

- Mango coconut smoothie for dessert

**Snack:** Sliced apple with peanut butter

## Day 8:

**Breakfast:** Whole grain toast with avocado spread

**Lunch:** Shrimp and vegetable stir-fry with low-sodium soy sauce

**Dinner:** Baked chicken thighs with rosemary and garlic

**Snack:** Celery sticks with cream cheese

## Day 9:

**Breakfast:** Greek yogurt parfait with granola and sliced strawberries

- Green tea

**Lunch:** Vegetable and lentil curry

- Basmati rice

**Dinner:** Baked tilapia with lemon and herbs

- Roasted Brussels sprouts

**Snack:** Chia seed pudding with mango

## Day 10:

**Breakfast:** Whole grain bagel with smoked salmon and cream cheese

- Orange juice

**Lunch:** Turkey and vegetable kebabs

**Dinner:** Grilled portobello mushrooms with balsamic glaze

**Snack:** Fresh pineapple chunks

## Day 11:

**Breakfast:** Spinach and mushroom frittata

**Lunch:** Quinoa salad with cucumber and mint

*Dinner:* Sweet potato mash

- Broccoli and cauliflower medley

*Snack:* Rice cake with almond butter and banana slices

## Day 12:

*Breakfast:* Smoothie with kale, pineapple, and coconut water

*Lunch:* Grilled chicken breast

*Dinner:* Stir-fried tofu with snow peas and carrots

*Snack:* Cottage cheese with sliced peaches

## Day 13:

*Breakfast:* Overnight oats with almond milk, chia seeds, and mixed berries

- Green tea

*Lunch:* Lentil and vegetable soup

- Whole grain roll

*Dinner:* Baked turkey cutlets with a cranberry glaze

- Steamed green beans

*Snack:* Greek yogurt with a drizzle of honey

## Day 14:

**Breakfast:** Whole grain pancakes with sliced bananas and a sprinkle of cinnamon

- Fresh orange segments

**Lunch:** Shrimp and avocado salad with a lime vinaigrette

**Dinner:** Roasted sweet potato wedges

- Grilled zucchini

**Snack:** Mixed berry smoothie with a touch of flaxseed

This meal plan is designed to provide a variety of nutrients while considering the dietary restrictions associated with CKD Stage 4. Portion sizes and specific food choices can be adjusted based on individual needs and preferences.

# Conclusion

In conclusion, the CKD Stage 4 Cookbook for Seniors serves as a comprehensive guide to not only managing but thriving with Chronic Kidney Disease. This well-designed cookbook offers a wide variety of meals that are intended to benefit individuals with Stage 4 CKD by fusing delectable flavors with nutritious ingredients that are kind to the kidneys. Everything from tasty lunch and dinner recipes to well-chosen breakfast options is attentively prepared to meet the unique dietary requirements associated with this stage of kidney illness.

Recognizing the need of nutrient management, the cookbook places a strong emphasis on meals that are low in sodium, mindful of phosphorus, and adjusted in potassium to help stop additional kidney damage. The meal plans are designed to help seniors with Stage 4 CKD manage their symptoms, maintain their general health, and improve their quality of life through balanced eating.

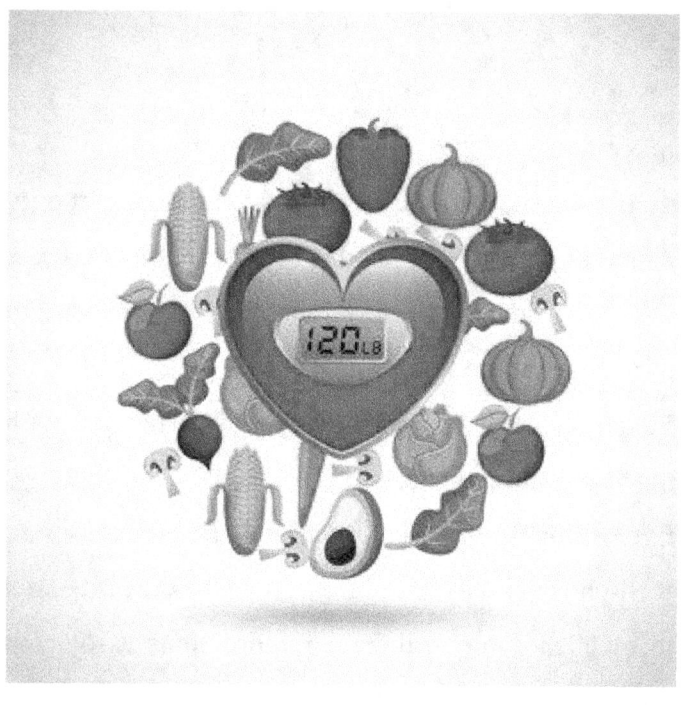

Beyond the enticing meals, this cookbook promotes a conscious approach to health by encouraging moderation in protein intake, regular monitoring of important indicators, and mindfulness regarding hydration intake. Working together with medical experts is still crucial to make sure that the meal plans follow specific dietary guidelines and medical recommendations.

For many readers, adopting this cookbook means taking back control of their health and wellbeing, not just managing Stage 4 CKD. Every recipe is a chance to enjoy the delight of flavorful, kidney-friendly food while also providing nourishment for the body. You're not only starting down the path to better kidney health when you embrace and adjust to this diet, but you're also cultivating a fresh sense of energy and harmony in your life. Your dedication to these dietary adjustments represents a significant financial investment in your well-being and the possibility of a more optimistic, lively future.

Keep in mind that every delicious meal is a step toward wellness, a self-care act that reflects a strong dedication to being a happier, healthier version of yourself.

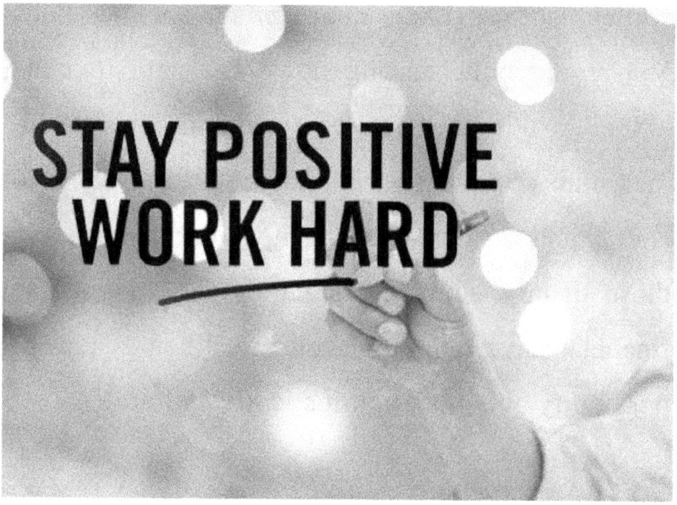
STAY POSITIVE
WORK HARD

# Weekly Meal Planner

# Journal

## Weekly Meal Planner Journal

Dates:

|  | BREAKFAST | LUNCH | DINNER | SNACKS |
|---|---|---|---|---|
| MON | | | | |
| TUE | | | | |
| WED | | | | |
| THU | | | | |
| FRI | | | | |
| SAT | | | | |
| SUN | | | | |

Shopping list

## NOTES

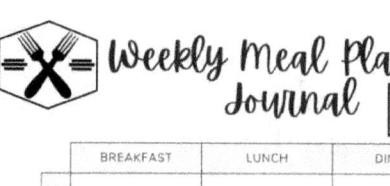

# Weekly Meal Planner Journal

Dates:

| | BREAKFAST | LUNCH | DINNER | SNACKS |
|---|---|---|---|---|
| MON | | | | |
| TUE | | | | |
| WED | | | | |
| THU | | | | |
| FRI | | | | |
| SAT | | | | |
| SUN | | | | |

Shopping list

_____
_____
_____
_____
_____
_____

**NOTES**

 **Weekly Meal Planner Journal**

Dates:

| | BREAKFAST | LUNCH | DINNER | SNACKS |
|---|---|---|---|---|
| MON | | | | |
| TUE | | | | |
| WED | | | | |
| THU | | | | |
| FRI | | | | |
| SAT | | | | |
| SUN | | | | |

Shopping list

**NOTES**

 **Weekly Meal Planner Journal**

Dates:

| | BREAKFAST | LUNCH | DINNER | SNACKS |
|---|---|---|---|---|
| MON | | | | |
| TUE | | | | |
| WED | | | | |
| THU | | | | |
| FRI | | | | |
| SAT | | | | |
| SUN | | | | |

Shopping list

**NOTES**

# Weekly Meal Planner Journal

Dates:

| | BREAKFAST | LUNCH | DINNER | SNACKS |
|---|---|---|---|---|
| MON | | | | |
| TUE | | | | |
| WED | | | | |
| THU | | | | |
| FRI | | | | |
| SAT | | | | |
| SUN | | | | |

Shopping list

**NOTES**

 **Weekly Meal Planner**
**Journal**

|  | BREAKFAST | LUNCH | DINNER | SNACKS |
|---|---|---|---|---|
| MON |  |  |  |  |
| TUE |  |  |  |  |
| WED |  |  |  |  |
| THU |  |  |  |  |
| FRI |  |  |  |  |
| SAT |  |  |  |  |
| SUN |  |  |  |  |

Shopping list

**NOTES**

www.ingramcontent.com/pod-product-compliance
Lightning Source LLC
Chambersburg PA
CBHW071057290526
45795CB00004B/1538